Christa McAuliffe Middle School
Library Media Center
16650 South Post Oak
Houston, Texas 77053

CONTENTS

Increase your physical activity 4

Before you begin an exercise program 7

Ready, set, go. 9

How are you doing? 18

Advice for women
with special conditions 22

Staying motivated. 28

Weekly activity log 30

Monthly progress rec   32

Cover and inte   s on pages 5, 8, 9, 17, 21, 29: Digital Imagery © copyright
2001 PhotoDi   es 11, 12, 14, 15, 16: © 2001 Rudolph King Studios;
page 30: © C   ion.

SECTION 1

INCREASE YOUR PHYSICAL ACTIVITY

Adding physical activity to your life doesn't mean you have to wear a sweat suit every day. Simple modifications to your lifestyle will help.

Even routine household chores can burn calories and help improve your health, although not at the same level as a structured exercise program. (See "Physical activity vs. exercise," below.)

The fact is that physical inactivity significantly increases your risk of heart disease and other health problems. But you can gain health benefits from doing moderate-intensity physical activity for just 30 minutes a day. You can even break these into several short sessions that add up to 30 minutes: for example, 10 minutes three times a day.

The key is attitude. Just pick something you like to do. Make a date with your spouse to go dancing every Friday. Go walking with a friend. Ride a bike with your grandchild.

And you'll gain even more health benefits if you have a regular, structured exercise program. It's never too late to start. This booklet offers you a simple plan for making fitness part of your everyday life so you look good and feel good.

PHYSICAL ACTIVITY VS. EXERCISE

- **Physical activity** is any body movement that burns calories, such as washing dishes, making the bed or walking your dog. (See "Every move counts" on page 6.)
- **Exercise** is a form of physical activity that involves a series of repetitive movements designed to strengthen or develop some part of the body. This includes sports such as swimming or running or an exercise plan like the one described on page 9.

Fitness pays
More than two-thirds of American adults don't get the recommended amount of exercise. Physical inactivity is more common among women than men. Yet physical activity — combined with eating well — is the key to improving your overall health and preventing illness. Regular exercise can:

- Help prevent coronary artery disease and stroke
- Reduce high blood pressure
- Prevent bone loss and osteoporosis
- Help improve coordination and balance, reducing the risk of injury from falls
- Help prevent and control type 2 diabetes by lowering blood sugar
- Help reduce your risk of certain cancers, such as colon, endometrial and breast cancers
- Help control weight and prevent obesity when combined with a healthy diet
- Help motivate you to cut down or quit smoking
- Help relieve mild to moderate depression and some forms of anxiety
- Increase energy level and decrease stress

Exercising regularly and staying physically active can help prevent or delay some diseases and disabilities as you grow older. In some cases it can improve your health if you already have a disease or a disability.

Are you fit? Probably not, if you sit most of the day. Other signs that you're not fit include:

- Feeling tired most of the time
- Being unable to keep up with others your age
- Avoiding physical activity because you tire quickly
- Becoming short of breath or tired when walking a short distance

These signs and symptoms can also occur because of heart problems or other diseases. If there's no medical explanation for the signs and symptoms, increasing your activity level will help you improve your physical condition.

EVERY MOVE COUNTS

You get greater health benefits with higher-intensity activities that last 30 minutes or more. But low- to moderate-intensity activities can complement your physical routine.

Here are some simple ways to increase your daily activity:

- Sweep your floors, patio and front walk every day.
- Instead of sitting and talking with a friend, go for a walk while you talk.
- Mow the grass (using a riding lawn mower doesn't count).
- Rake leaves, prune bushes or dig in the garden.
- Go out for a short walk before breakfast.
- Walk or bike to the store instead of driving.
- When watching TV, use a stationary bike.
- Walk the dog.
- Park farther away at the shopping mall and walk the extra distance. While you're shopping, walk around the entire mall a couple of times.
- Avoid drive-throughs. Park the car and walk in.
- Don't use the closest bathroom. Use one that requires you to walk a bit.
- Set a timer to remind yourself to get up and stretch or walk around the house or office.
- If you're waiting for an airplane or a table at a restaurant, take a walk.
- Take the stairs instead of an elevator.

To learn how to gauge the intensity of your activities, see "How are you doing?" on page 16.

SECTION 2

BEFORE YOU BEGIN AN EXERCISE PROGRAM

See your doctor before starting an exercise program if you're a woman over age 50 (or a man over age 40) and you haven't been exercising on a regular basis. The same applies if you smoke, are overweight or have a chronic health problem, such as:

- Cardiovascular disease
- High blood pressure
- Osteoporosis
- Kidney disease
- Liver disease
- Arthritis

In addition to determining if you're medically ready to exercise, your doctor can explain the specific benefits. Ask what exercises are appropriate for you. And, together, set performance and outcome goals.

Also check with your doctor if:

- You become lightheaded or have discomfort in your chest during exercise.
- You have more shortness of breath than others your age doing the same activity.
- You tire easily from mild exertion.

If you're taking medications, ask your doctor if this affects how and when you exercise and what types of exercise you can do. Exercise can affect how your body reacts to some medications. For example, if you have diabetes, exercise can lower your blood sugar. As a result, you may require a lower amount of insulin or other diabetes medication.

Everyday Fitness: Look Good, Feel Good

REDUCING THE RISKS OF EXERCISE

Most risks of exercise stem from doing too much, too vigorously, with too little previous activity. To reduce risks:

1. **Begin gradually.** Don't overdo it. If you have trouble talking to a companion during your workout, you're probably pushing too hard.
2. **Stretch.** Proper stretching actually lengthens the muscle tissue, making it less tight and therefore less prone to trauma and tears. Start slowly and hold your stretch at least 15 to 30 seconds, with a minimum of three repetitions for each stretch. Don't bounce. And don't stretch cold muscles — it can strain and irritate the tissue. Warm up first. Walk before you jog, and jog before you run. It's actually best to stretch *after* you exercise when your muscles are heated by increased blood flow and more flexible.
3. **Exercise regularly but moderately.** Never exercise to the point of nausea, dizziness or severe shortness of breath. Other red flags include heart palpitations, tightness in your chest, or pain in your chest, arm or jaw. If you experience any of these signs and symptoms, stop exercising and get immediate medical care. They may indicate a more serious medical problem.
4. **Drink plenty of water to prevent dehydration.** Drink two cups of water about 2 hours before working out and one-half cup every 15 to 20 minutes while exercising. Don't rely on your thirst to tell you when you need a drink. When you exercise, your thirst mechanism is suppressed.
5. **Always cool down.** Slow your activity down before you stop and then finish with stretching. This reduces stress on your heart as well as your muscles.

SECTION 3

Ready, set, go

You get health benefits from simply being more active during the day. However, a regular, structured exercise program gives you maximum benefits. An optimal exercise plan incorporates aerobic, strength and balance, and flexibility exercises.

Aerobic. These activities increase your breathing and heart rate to improve the health of your heart, lung and circulatory system. Having more endurance also improves your stamina for the tasks you need to do every day — such as doing household chores and climbing stairs.

Strength and balance. These exercises build stronger muscles to improve posture, balance and coordination. Strength exercises also increase your metabolism, which helps keep your weight in check.

Flexibility. Stretching before and after an activity helps increase the range to which you can bend and stretch joints, muscles and ligaments. Flexibility helps prevent joint pain and injury.

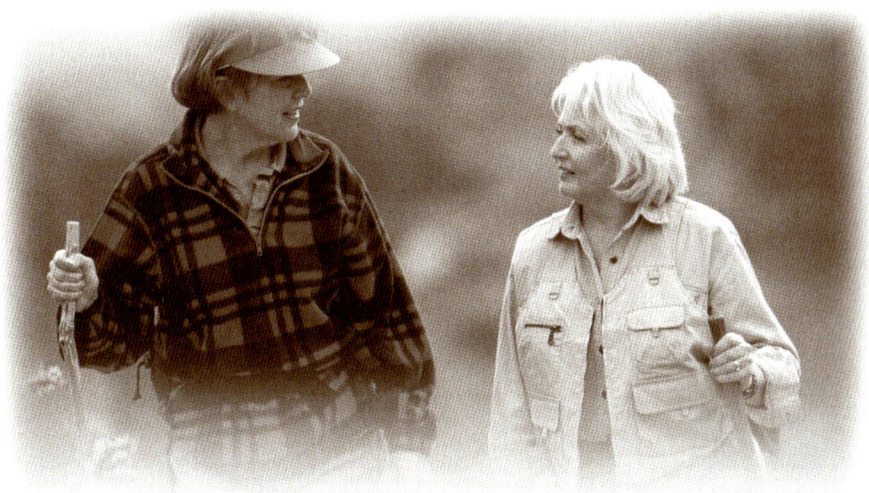

Everyday Fitness: Look Good, Feel Good 9

Getting started
Now you're ready to get started. Pick something you think is fun — you'll be more likely to stick with it. Here are some other tips to help you stay on track:

- **Set your sights on 6 months.** People who stick with a new behavior for at least 6 months usually have long-term success — it becomes a habit.
- **Join a class.** Many health clubs now offer classes for people not used to exercising. Ask about the type of exercises involved and the intensity.
- **Enjoy the exercise.** Make your goal the exercise itself, rather than limiting it to a goal like losing weight.
- **Be patient with yourself.** Improvements will occur if you're consistent with your exercise.

A sample exercise plan
Here's an exercise plan that's safe for almost anyone, regardless of age or fitness level.

Warm-up (5 to 10 minutes). Begin each exercise session by warming up. Walk slowly, then increase your pace until you feel warm. Warming up your muscles reduces your risk of injury.

Flexibility exercises (5 to 10 minutes). Stretches should be gentle and slow. Don't bounce. Stretch only until you feel a slight tension in the muscle. Continue to breathe normally while stretching.

Here are four types of stretches. Do at least three repetitions of each one.

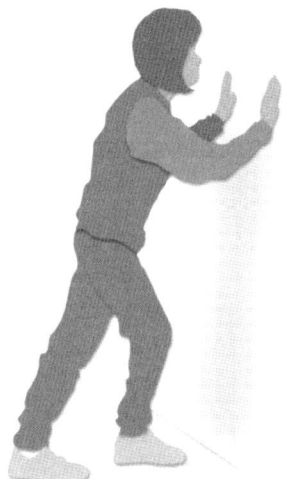

- **Calf stretch** (see left). Stand at arm's length from the wall. Place one leg forward with the knee bent. Keep your other leg back with knee straight and heel down. Keeping your back straight, move your hips toward the wall until you feel a stretch in the calf of your extended leg. Keep both heels on the ground. Hold for 15 to 30 seconds. Relax. Repeat with the other leg.

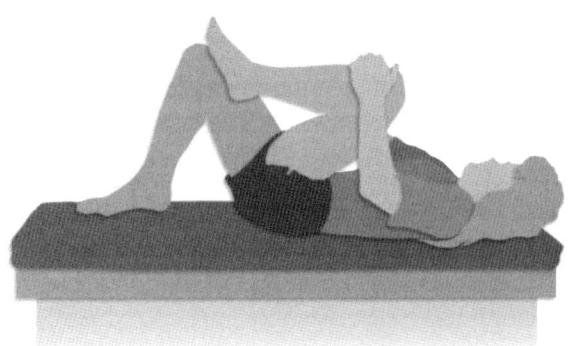

- **Lower back stretch** (see above). Lie on a firm surface (floor or table) with your hips and knees bent and feet flat on the surface. Pull your left knee toward your shoulder with both hands. If you have knee problems, pull from the back of your thigh. Hold for 15 to 30 seconds. Relax. Repeat with your other leg.

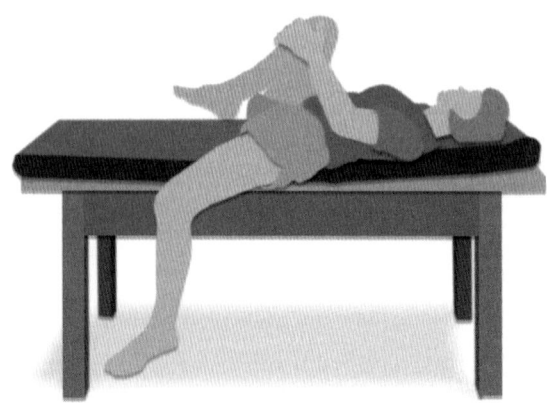

- **Upper thigh stretch** (see above). Lie on your back on a table or firm bed, with one leg and hip as safely near the edge as possible. Grasp the knee of the other leg with both hands and pull toward your chest until your lower back flattens against the table. If you have knee problems, pull from the back of your thigh. Then relax your straight leg so it hangs over the edge. Hold for 15 to 30 seconds. Relax. Repeat with the opposite leg.

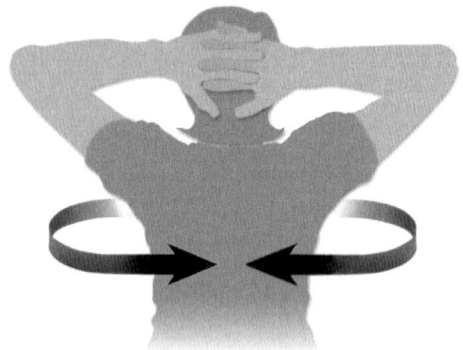

- **Chest stretch** (see left). Clasp your hands behind your head. Pull your elbows gently back by pinching your shoulder blades together while inhaling deeply. Hold position for 15 to 30 seconds, while breathing normally. Relax.

Aerobic activity (30 minutes). Aim for 30 minutes of moderately intense activity. Some examples include walking briskly, golfing (walk don't ride), raking leaves, playing badminton or tennis, bike riding, mowing the lawn with a push mower, social dancing and swimming.

To build up to 30 minutes, start with 10 minutes and increase your time by 5-minute increments over several weeks. (For more information about pacing yourself, see "Don't ignore pain" on page 15.)

Strength and balance exercises (10 to 20 minutes). Add strength and balance exercises to your routine at least twice a week. Do strength and balance exercises separately if you prefer. Just be sure to include warm-up, stretching and cool-down as part of the session. Start with 10 to 12 repetitions and work up to 20.

Remember to move slowly. If you do the exercise too quickly, you may strain a muscle. (For more information on the benefits of strength training, see page 14.)

On the next two pages you'll find four strength and balance exercises to try, but check with your doctor first if you have health conditions such as arthritis.

STRENGTH AND BALANCE EXERCISES: BREATHE PROPERLY

For most of the following strength and balance exercises, breathe out and through your mouth during the first part of the movement, counting slowly to four. Then breathe in through your nose, counting slowly to four on the second part of the movement. But breathing recommendations for heel raises (see page 13) are different: Breath in, do the heel raise while slightly exhaling, then breath in on the way down.

Everyday Fitness: Look Good, Feel Good

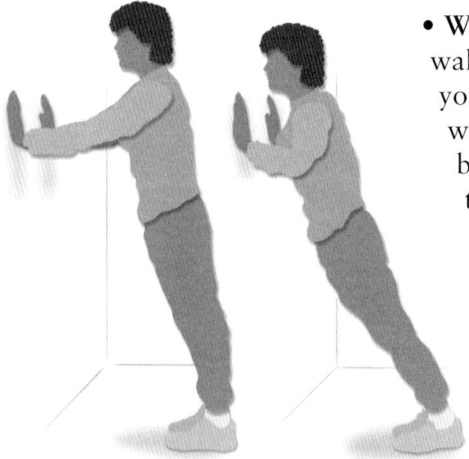

- **Wall push-ups** (see left). Face the wall and stand far enough away so you can place your palms on the wall with your elbows slightly bent. Keeping your heels flat on the floor, slowly bend your elbows and lean toward the wall, supporting your weight with your arms. Straighten your arms and return to an upright position. For increased resistance (and as balance allows), try standing farther from the wall. Increase the number of repetitions as your muscles become stronger. This exercise can also help prevent cramps in calf muscles.

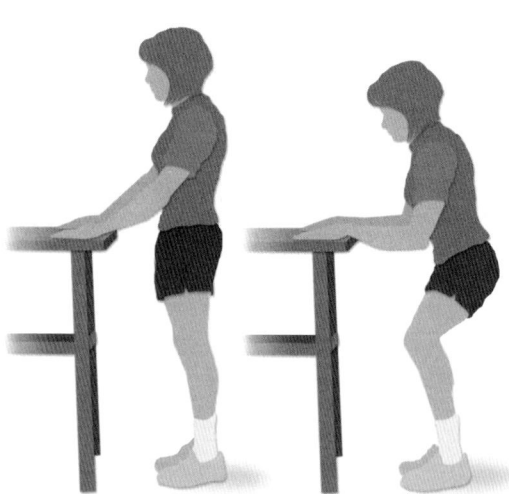

- **Standing squats** (see left). Stand with your feet flat on the floor, slightly more than shoulder-width apart, toes pointed ahead or slightly outward. Keeping your back straight and looking straight ahead, slowly lower your hips downward and backward as you bend your knees anywhere from 30 degrees to 60 degrees. Pause for a second and then return to your starting position. To maintain balance, lightly hold on to a table or countertop in front of you with one hand. You may also want to place a chair behind you for added safety. Increase the number of repetitions as your muscles become stronger.

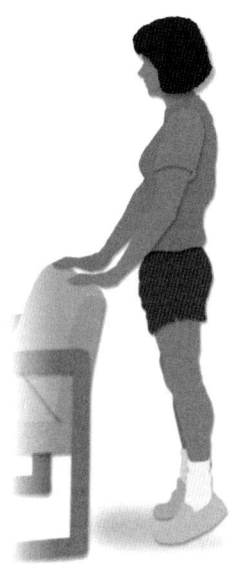

- **Heel raises** (see left). Stand with your feet flat on the floor (about 12 inches apart), holding on to the back of a sturdy chair. Slowly raise your heels and stand on tiptoe. Hold the position for a couple of seconds. Then slowly lower your heels back down. Increase repetitions as your muscles become stronger. To improve balance, try the exercise holding on to the chair with only one finger, then without using hands.

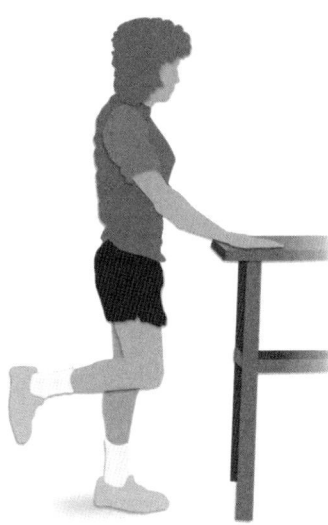

- **Leg lifts** (see left). Stand with your feet flat on the floor (about 12 inches apart), holding on to a table or the back of a sturdy chair for balance. Slowly bend one knee so your foot lifts up behind you, without moving your spine. Hold the position. Slowly lower your foot all the way back down. Repeat with the other leg. To improve balance, try the exercise holding on to the chair or table with only one finger, then without using hands.

Cool down (5 to 10 minutes). End each exercise session by walking slowly. You may also repeat the same stretching exercises you did earlier.

WHY SHOULD YOU DO STRENGTH EXERCISES?

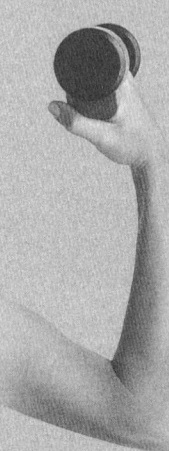

Muscle mass diminishes with age. Between the ages of 30 and 70, you'll lose about 1 percent of your muscle strength each year, primarily through inactivity. Losing lean muscle mass doesn't just affect your strength. It affects your balance and diminishes your energy.

You don't have to be a body builder to see benefits. Challenging your muscles with strengthening exercises for as little as 20 minutes twice weekly can improve your well-being. Regular strength training helps to:

- **Increase strength and stability.** You're never too old to benefit. A study involving 100 nursing home residents, ages 72 to 98, found that 10 weeks of progressive strength training for thigh and lower leg muscles increased muscle strength an average of 113 percent. Walking speed and stair climbing also improved.
- **Maintain and increase bone mineral density.** When bone is stressed appropriately through muscle movement, it gets stronger. In one study of postmenopausal women, half of the participants lifted weights twice a week. One year later, those women had increased their muscle mass an average of 9 percent and the bone density in their hips and spine by 1 percent. By contrast, the women who didn't lift weights experienced a decrease in bone density of about 2 percent.
- **Control body fat by boosting your metabolic rate.** When you lose muscle, your body gradually becomes less efficient at burning calories. That's because muscle burns more calories than fat does. So the more muscle mass your body has, the more calories it will burn, even when you're at rest.

DON'T IGNORE PAIN

You may be enthusiastic about starting to exercise. However, it's important to start at a manageable level and gradually work your way up. If you do too much too quickly, you can injure yourself. Below are some helpful tips for treating minor injuries, but call your doctor for advice if the injury is serious:

- **Rest.** Don't keep pushing yourself if you feel pain. Exercise injuries usually heal if you stop activities that aggravate the condition. Yet, resting doesn't necessarily mean stopping exercise altogether. In some cases, you can switch to a different type of exercise that won't aggravate your injury.
- **Treat the pain.** Apply cold to an injury for the first 48 hours to help relieve pain and swelling. After 48 hours use cold or heat or a combination of both to relieve pain. You can also take acetaminophen (Tylenol, generics) or a non-steroidal anti-inflammatory drug, such as aspirin or ibuprofen (Advil, Motrin), unless your doctor advises otherwise.
- **Protect the injury.** One way to reduce pain is to wrap the injury with a stretchy bandage. This may reduce swelling and decrease pain signals from the injured area. Bandaging will also remind you to avoid movements that may aggravate the injury. Don't wrap it too tightly or you'll impair circulation.

SECTION 4

How are you doing?

These three tests will help you assess how fit you are right now, before you start an exercise program. After that, do them every month to compare the results and see your progress. To record your results, use the "Monthly progress record" on page 30. Remember to check with your doctor before you do these tests if necessary. (See "Before you begin an exercise program" on page 5.)

1. **Endurance.** See how far you can walk in 6 minutes. Write down the distance (feet, blocks, laps or miles). Do this test every month. As your endurance improves, you should find that you walk farther.

ASSEMBLE YOUR EQUIPMENT

Your equipment can be as simple as appropriate athletic shoes and a few common household items, such as homemade weights and a nonslip chair.

Make your own weights by filling old socks with beans or pennies, or by partially filling a half-gallon milk jug with water or sand. Or buy used weights at an athletic equipment store or through newspaper classified ads.

If you have a health problem, check with your doctor or physical therapist first to determine what equipment is right for you. Here are some tips on buying exercise equipment:

- **Consider your goals.** What do you want to accomplish? Are you looking to build strength, increase flexibility, improve endurance? Your equipment should address your personal needs.
- **Try equipment before you buy it.** If you have access to a health club or if your friends have any in-home equipment, try out their equipment to find out what interests you the

2. **Strength.** The chair-stand test measures your progress in lower-body strength. Use a chair that's pushed against the wall so it won't move. Count the number of times you can smoothly move from a sitting to a standing position in 30 seconds, without using your hands. Record the number of times. Your count should increase each month.
3. **Balance.** Time yourself as you stand on one foot (without support) for as long as possible. Record your time. Repeat the test while standing on the other foot. Your time should increase each month. *Note:* Stand near a sturdy chair while you're doing this. If you lose your balance, you can steady yourself with the chair.

most. Or go to a fitness equipment store in your workout gear and try out different pieces. Your goal is to find something you will likely use regularly. Some equipment, such as ski machines, which work your arms and legs, may require time to learn, but can be well worth the effort.

- **Realize that one machine isn't going to do it all.** Most exercise equipment works on specific body parts, not the entire body. You can buy just one piece of equipment, but be sure to include other activities in your workout. For example, if you buy a treadmill, be sure to do stretching and strengthening exercises as well. Be wary of gimmicks — no device will give you easy or effortless results.
- **Know your space.** Be sure you have proper floor space, electrical outlets, ventilation and lighting.
- **Research your options.** Check out fitness and consumer magazines that rate exercise equipment. Visit stores with knowledgeable salespeople and ask questions about safety and reliability. And be sure to check the fine print before you buy anything. Read the details on warranties, delivery and return policies.

AVERAGE CALORIES BURNED*

You can use this chart as an approximate guide for determining the average number of calories you may burn with 10 minutes of continuous activity.

ACTIVITY (10 minutes continuous)	YOUR WEIGHT		
	120-130 pounds	160-170 pounds	190-200 pounds
Walking (normal or treadmill)			
2 mph (30 min/mile)	30	40	45
3 mph (20 min/mile)	40	50	60
4 mph (15 min/mile)	55	70	85
Aerobic dance	60-105	75-140	90-165
Bicycling			
Outdoor	40-145	50-195	60-230
Stationary	25-145	30-195	40-230
Bowling	30-40	40-50	45-60
Calisthenics	40-105	50-140	60-165
Dancing	30-80	40-105	45-120
Jogging			
5 mph (12 min/mile)	90	115	135
6 mph (10 min/mile)	105	140	165
Skiing			
Cross-country	60-145	75-195	90-230
Downhill	40-90	50-115	60-135
Swimming	50-125	65-165	75-200
Tennis	50-95	65-130	75-150

*The number of calories you burn can vary a great deal, depending on the intensity and duration of activity as well as your body weight and composition. The longer you exercise, the more calories you'll burn. And if you weigh 175 pounds you'll use more energy walking 30 minutes than a 120-pound person will.

HOW HARD ARE YOU WORKING?

The Perceived Exertion Scale is also called the Borg Scale, named after the scientist who developed it. Below you'll find a modified version. This tool helps describe how hard you feel you're working during a particular activity. How much effort do you put into it? How much physical stress and fatigue do you experience?

For the activity to produce health benefits, you need to exert a moderate to somewhat strong effort. That means you'll need a 3 or 4 on the modified scale below. A zero rating indicates a minimal level of exertion, such as sitting comfortably in a chair, while a 10 corresponds to a maximal effort, like jogging up a steep hill.

If you've been inactive and are out of condition, don't push it. (See "Reducing the risks of exercise" on page 8.) Gradually increase the intensity and duration to reach your goal. The longer you keep at it, the more you'll be able to do.

Perceived Exertion Scale (Modified)

Rate yourself using the scale below. What level of exertion do you feel during a specific physical activity? Pay attention to how your entire body feels, not just a certain part.

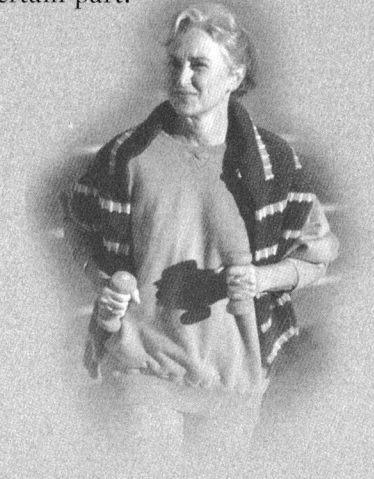

0 Nothing at all
1 Very weak
2 Weak
3 Moderate
4 Somewhat strong
5 Strong
6 Stronger
7 Very strong
8 More difficult
9 Very difficult
10 Extremely difficult

SECTION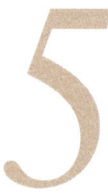

ADVICE FOR WOMEN WITH SPECIAL CONDITIONS

Traditionally, people with certain chronic conditions were discouraged from exercising. But researchers have found that exercise can actually improve some chronic conditions in many people. Exercise also provides stress relief and acts as a natural antidepressant.

Chronic diseases are illnesses that are prolonged and usually can't be cured. But they often can be effectively managed with healthy lifestyle choices, medication and other treatments. They include, for example, arthritis, asthma, coronary artery disease, diabetes and osteoporosis.

Here are some basic guidelines for exercising with specific chronic diseases. *If you have a chronic condition, talk to your doctor about an exercise program that's appropriate for you.* Let your doctor know if your symptoms get better or worse, which might warrant a change in your exercise program.

ARTHRITIS

Although pain and stiffness may discourage you from activity, using joints during regular appropriate exercise may actually reduce pain and injury. It can improve your energy level and your ability to accomplish daily tasks and activities. And the fact that exercise helps you control your weight is especially important. This helps you avoid placing unnecessary stress on your joints.

Any movement, no matter how little, can help. Choose low-impact activities. Water exercises are ideal because water buoyancy takes weight off your joints. Swimming laps, water walking or jogging, and water aerobics are examples.

Other forms of low-impact exercise that place less stress on joints include biking, cross-country skiing, stair-steppers and snowshoeing.

Let comfort be your guide when exercising with arthritis. To help:

- *Go easy.* Start gradually and don't overdo it. If you have severe pain, stop that particular exercise. Don't exercise tender, injured or badly inflamed joints.
- *Warm up first.* Warm up muscles and joints with a heating pad, massage or by gently walking in place for a few minutes. A warm bath or shower before you exercise may also help.
- *Try different times of the day.* Exercise at the time of day you feel the least pain and stiffness.
- *Take a pain reliever.* Unless your doctor suggests otherwise, take a nonsteroidal anti-inflammatory drug, such as aspirin or ibuprofen, 1 hour before exercising to limit swelling and reduce pain.
- *Avoid bouncing and high-impact exercise.* Slow stretching can increase a stiff joint's range of motion. Don't bounce as you stretch. Avoid jumping and stop-and-start exercises. If you're having a flare-up, focus on other joints.

ASTHMA

Exercise is a common trigger of asthma symptoms. This is called exercise-induced asthma (EIA). You're more prone to EIA if you have asthma with allergies. Signs and symptoms of EIA include:

- Coughing
- Wheezing
- Chest tightness
- Shortness of breath

It's important to know the difference between EIA and being out of condition. Someone who is fit usually will only experience these symptoms with vigorous activity or exercise. If you're out of condition, you may experience these symptoms even at low levels of exertion.

But you don't have to be inactive if you have asthma. In fact, it's best if you're physically active. Regular exercise strengthens your heart and lungs, so they don't have to work so hard to expel air. It also helps you lose weight, so you can breathe easier.

Hear are some valuable tips:

- Inhale bronchodilator medications, such as albuterol, 15 to 30 minutes before exercising to help prevent symptoms.
- Do 5 to 10 minutes of warm-up stretching or light exercise before vigorous activity to help relax and open your airways.
- Choose activities that are less likely to trigger asthma symptoms. For example, swimming (involving warm, humid air) is often handled well.
- Choose activities that involve short or intermittent periods of exercise, such as golf, walking, volleyball or softball.
- Be aware that cold-air activities, such as skiing or ice hockey, are more likely to cause wheezing. If you do exercise in cold weather, wear a face mask to warm the air you breathe. Don't exercise in temperatures below zero.
- Be aware that other aerobic sports, such as distance running, soccer or basketball, can trigger symptoms.
- Consult your doctor before starting an exercise program. Together you can plan a program that will work for you.

Above all, don't let asthma prevent you from maintaining an active life. Several Olympic athletes with asthma have gone on to win gold medals.

CORONARY ARTERY DISEASE

Regular exercise helps your heart pump blood more efficiently, improves your cholesterol levels and may lower your blood pressure.

Doctors often recommend exercise for people who have had a heart attack as part of their cardiac rehabilitation program. In fact, a recent study shows that regular exercise helps reduce the risk of a second heart attack and an untimely death.

You may worry about having a heart attack during exercise. However, most heart attacks occur during rest — not activity. Of people who have heart attacks during strenuous exertion, most are sedentary, have underlying heart disease and overdo it. To minimize risk and maximize benefits of exercise, follow these tips:

- *Exercise regularly.* Cardiovascular risk increases if you alternate intense workouts with weeks to months of inactivity.
- *Exercise, don't compete.* Avoid physical and emotional intensity in competitive sports.
- *Wait 2 to 3 hours after a large meal before exercising.* Digestion directs blood to your digestive system and away from your heart.
- *Take the talk test.* If you can talk easily while exercising, you're probably not overexerting yourself.
- *Don't walk near heavy traffic.* Carbon monoxide pollution reduces oxygen to your heart.
- *Listen to your body.* If you experience heart palpitations, lightheadedness, or pain in your chest, jaw or arm, stop exercising and call your doctor.
- *Cool down gradually.* This puts less stress on your heart. Slowly taper off your exercise intensity until your heart rate has returned to normal.

DIABETES

Exercise can lower blood sugar and increase insulin efficiency, improving blood sugar control. It also helps prevent or delay the development of cardiovascular disease — the leading cause of death for people with diabetes.

However, your activity must be planned to fit your mealtimes and medication dosage. If you're taking oral diabetic medications or insulin, eat a small snack before exercising if it's been more than an hour since you last ate. As a rule, a high-carbohydrate snack (such as a glass of juice, crackers or fruit) is good before or during mild to moderate exercise.

Check your blood sugar before and after exercising. If it's under 70 mg/dL, you may need to eat a snack to avoid low blood sugar. Don't exercise if your blood sugar level is above 300 mg/dL. Once you establish a regular exercise program, your doctor may need to lower the amount of insulin or oral medication you take.

If your blood sugar control is poor or if you have diabetic eye disease (retinopathy) or blood vessel problems, ask your doctor which activities are safe for you.

EXERCISE AND BREAST CANCER TREATMENT

A recent study shows that regular, moderate exercise helps maintain strength and control weight gain during treatment following breast cancer surgery.

If you're receiving chemotherapy or radiation, your treatment may leave you feeling tired, anxious, sick or depressed. You may worry about overexertion. But inactivity usually makes people feel worse.

Walking and other forms of moderately intense exercise can help you feel better both physically and mentally. Not only can regular exercise help you cope with cancer, it can also give you a greater sense of control over your life.

Before you get started, talk with your doctor about what exercise program is best for you.

> ## EXERCISE AND DEPRESSION
>
> Studies show that increased aerobic exercise or strength training helps relieve symptoms of depression. From a physical standpoint, exercise heats up your body and decreases muscle tension. Some researchers suggest that exercise changes neurochemical activity in the brain, helping to elevate your mood.
>
> A regular exercise program can also provide you with a chance for more social interaction and support, not to mention a sense of accomplishment as you build strength and endurance.
>
> Moderate exercise is the key — overtraining may actually cause symptoms that mimic depression.

OSTEOPOROSIS

Because of the varying degrees of osteoporosis and the risk of fracture, if you've been diagnosed with this bone-thinning disease, ask your doctor for advice on an exercise program that's safe and appropriate for you.

Regular exercise builds muscle and helps maintain, and possibly increase, bone density. By strengthening your muscles and bones and improving your balance, you can reduce the risk of falls and resulting fractures often associated with osteoporosis.

Combine strength exercises with weight-bearing exercise. Brisk walking is usually an ideal weight-bearing exercise because you can do it anywhere with minimal risk of injury. If walking is painful, try riding a stationary bike. However, this may be less effective because it's not a full weight-bearing exercise.

Avoid high-impact exercise that puts excessive stress on your bones, such as tennis or jogging. Avoid rowing machines — they require deep forward bending that may lead to a spine fracture. Stiffness the morning after exercise is normal. But, if joint, bone or muscle pain is severe or persists, see your doctor.

SECTION 6
STAYING MOTIVATED

Starting an exercise program takes initiative. Sticking with it takes commitment. You should see some results within weeks. You'll feel invigorated and your stamina will increase. To stay motivated:

- **Choose an activity that fits your personality and lifestyle.** No single form of aerobic exercise is best. Do you like to exercise alone or in a group? If you prefer solitude, walking may be your first choice. Or perhaps you'd like to walk with a friend or family member. If group activities appeal to you and motivate you, enroll in an aerobic dance class or water aerobics class. Do you like to be outdoors, or would you prefer to stay inside? To combat boredom, watch television or listen to tapes while you use indoor exercise equipment.
- **Fit exercise into your daily routine.** If it seems hard to find time to exercise, remember it only takes 30 minutes a day of aerobic activity to improve your fitness level greatly. Walk for half an hour during your child's music lesson. Swim before eating during your lunch hour. Be creative.
- **Vary your activities.** To keep things interesting, change your activity every once in a while. Walk one day. Swim another. Bike on the weekend. And if you need good weather for your exercise of choice, have a backup plan for rainy or snowy days (for example, walk in a mall instead of outdoors).
- **Learn a new sport or take lessons to brush up on one you know.** There are many new forms of physical activity that you may not have tried. How about learning to line dance, square dance or rollerskate? Or maybe your skills at an old favorite are rusty.

- **Set performance goals.** Start with simple goals, such as just doing the exercise occasionally. Once you've started, set performance goals for the next 6 months. People who can stick with a new behavior for this length of time usually end up making it a habit.
- **Get your family involved.** You can support each other, and you'll be doing them a favor by helping them develop an important health habit.
- **If you stop, start again.** Don't lose hope if you lapse for some reason. Just get going again and gradually return to the level you were at before.

The benefits of exercise are beyond dispute. And the best part is you don't need to run a marathon to gain those benefits. With a little time and determination, you can be on your way to a healthier, more active life.

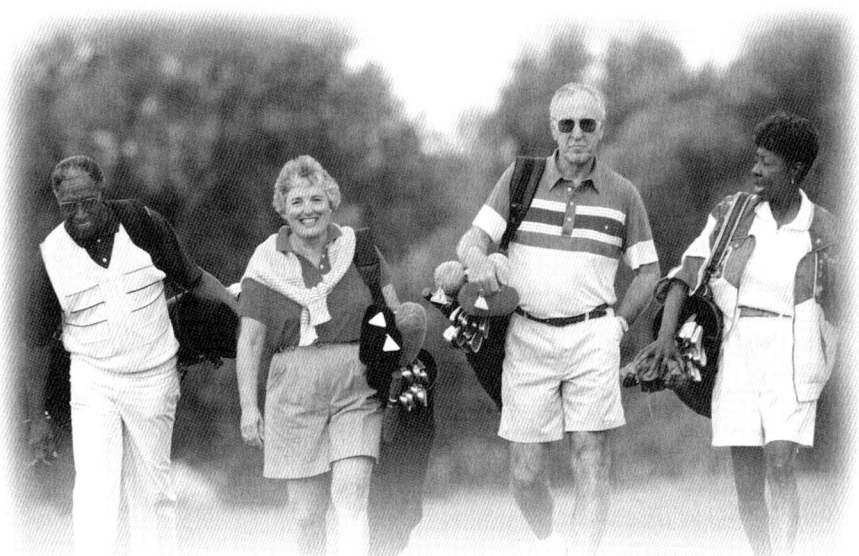

SECTION 7

WEEKLY ACTIVITY LOG

Make copies of this weekly log so you have enough for the whole year. Keep these performance goals in mind as you plan your week and document your time:

- **Aerobic activity.** 30 minutes a day (for a total of 3 1/2 hours a week)
- **Strength and balance exercise.** Twice a week
- **Stretching.** Include as part of every exercise session

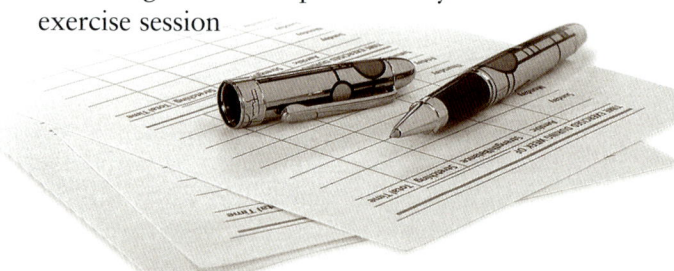

TIME EXERCISED DURING WEEK OF_____

	Aerobic	Strength/Balance	Stretching	Total Time
Sunday				
Monday				
Tuesday				
Wednesday				
Thursday				
Friday				
Saturday				

TIME EXERCISED DURING WEEK OF _____

	Aerobic	Strength/Balance	Stretching	Total Time
Sunday				
Monday				
Tuesday				
Wednesday				
Thursday				
Friday				
Saturday				

TIME EXERCISED DURING WEEK OF _____

	Aerobic	Strength/Balance	Stretching	Total Time
Sunday				
Monday				
Tuesday				
Wednesday				
Thursday				
Friday				
Saturday				

Everyday Fitness: Look Good, Feel Good

SECTION 8

MONTHLY PROGRESS RECORD

YEAR_____

Test your fitness on the same day each month for a year to track your progress.

	ENDURANCE	STRENGTH	BALANCE
	How far you walk in 6 minutes	How many times you sit/stand in 30 seconds	How long you can stand on each foot
JAN			
FEB			
MAR			
APR			
MAY			
JUN			
JUL			
AUG			
SEP			
OCT			
NOV			
DEC			

Chart adapted from *Exercise: A Guide from the National Institute on Aging*, National Institutes of Health, 1998.

GLOSSARY

Endometrial cancer: Cancer that develops in the lining of the uterus. It is usually curable if diagnosed early.

Exercise-induced asthma (EIA): Asthma triggered by exercise. Signs and symptoms may include coughing, wheezing, chest tightness and shortness of breath.

Metabolic rate: The rate at which your body is burning calories through the function of body processes.

Neurochemical activity: The chemical process of the nervous system.

Osteoporosis: Weakening of bones due to the loss of bone mineral content. Bones become less dense and more likely to break.

Type 2 diabetes: A disease characterized by poor blood sugar control due to the pancreas not making enough insulin, cells becoming resistant to insulin, or both.

INDEX

Calories
 burned in 10 minutes, 20

Equipment
 buying, 18-19
 homemade, 18
Exercise
 breast cancer treatment and, 26
 definition of, 4
 depression and, 27
 preparing for, 7
 reducing risks from, 8
 sample plan, 10
 special conditions and, 22-27
 starting, 10
 strength and balance, 13-15
 types of, 9, 13

Perceived exertion scale, 21
Physical activity, 4, 6

Stretches, 11-12

DATE DUE			

3 3396 01803400 2

613
EVE

**Everyday fitness :
look good, feel good**

CHRISTA MCAULIFFE M.S.

226044 01595 33339B 35298E   022

Christa McAuliffe Middle Schoo
Library Media Center
16650 South Post Oak
Houston, Texas 77053